Chasing the Skinny

LaNette

Chasing the Skinny, Transforming My Life Despite Adversity

LaNette Parson

Chasing the Skinny, LLC.

Bettendorf, IA 52722

www.chasingtheskinny.com

Ordering Information

Quantity sales: Special discounts are available on quantity purchases by corporations, associations, and others. For details, contact the publisher at the address above.

Orders by U.S. trade bookstores and wholesalers:

Please contact Chasing the Skinny, LLC Tel: 240-626-5566

www.chasingtheskinny.com

Social Media: @ChasingtheSkinny

ISBN-13: 978-1724370020

ISBN-10: 1724370022

Cover Design by Alicia Kenny

Edited by Ebony K. Matkins

Photo credit: Cheyenne Brown and Melissa Jakes

For Cymone

May you always feel like you are yourself
and you are enough! I love you for exactly
who you are and cannot wait to see who
you become! Love Mommy!

and

All the girls and women who never
thought they were skinny enough or slim
enough! God created you perfect in his
sight! Be exactly who God created you to
be!

Acknowledgment

Thank you, God! Without you, I am nothing! I may not be perfect but striving towards the mark and thank you for your son Jesus leaving a shining example!

Dante Turner, you are my everything! d there is no one else I would rather do life with than you! Thank for your constant motivation, support and being my rock! I fall in love with you more and more every day! #foreverturning

DeLois Moore, Mom I wrote a book! Thank you for always being a silent strong force! Thank you for setting an example for me and telling me to always have a plan! I love you so much!

Dr. Jiajoyce Conway, thank you for always being a phone call away! Thank you for believing in me when I didn't believe in myself and always having an encouraging word and a prayer! It's my book so I love you more!

Ebony Matkins who knew an 8-hour tour, 10 years ago would lead us here? Eb, you have supported me more times than I can count, you have been that calm steady voice in the middle of my storms. Thank you for editing my book and many more to come! We are Aggies and Sisters forever!

Alicia Kenny, thank you for designing my book cover, back cover, and logo because you believed in me. Your generosity will never be forgotten and always be appreciated.

So many people countless others to thank. Especially those who bought my book presales on a cover and my name! Your support is greatly appreciated!

Pamela Batty	Summer Blount
Kesha Brooks	Cheyenne Brown
Paris Bullock	Joy Champion
Troy Conway	Alteric Dunston
Norrine Harper	Melissa Jakes
Arthnise Lockhart	Nadine Martin
Ashlee McKinney	Sheila Parker
Tres Rahim	Deborah Rice
Pat Robinson	J Alden Smith
Cassandra Springer	Eleshia Thomas

Ingredients

Ingredients

Daily Affirmation

- I will achieve greatness
- Today, I am brimming with energy and overflowing with joy
- I love and accept myself for who I am
- My body is healthy; my mind is brilliant; my soul is tranquil
- I believe I can do all things through Christ that strengthen me
- Everything that is happening now is happening for my ultimate good
- I am the architect of my life; I build its foundation and choose its contents
- I forgive those who have harmed me in my past and peacefully detach from them
- My ability to conquer my challenges is limitless; my potential to succeed is infinite
- Today, I abandon my old habits embrace a new, positive, lifestyle

"If at first you don't succeed, try,
try, try again"

-W.E. Hickson

Chapter 1
Tried and Failed

You are about to find out the secret to my weight loss, that took me 20 years to figure out. I felt like a yoyo going up and down with my weight. For the majority of my life I have been a size 12, the smallest an 8 and the biggest a 16. I always convinced myself that 200 pounds was my scary weight. To my dismay in, April 2017 I weighed in at 240 pounds. Wasn't I supposed to be under 200 pounds? I mean according to my driver's license I was still 170 pounds...why would I dispute that and acknowledge what the scale clearly showed?

For 20+ years I have tried and failed to conform to society's definition of skinny. The Body Mass Index (BMI) for a woman of my size is 36.5. But I have hips and dips that BMI didn't account for. So, what are some of the fad diets I have tried? How much time do you have because there has been a plethora of them. I'll start with California company with the home based videos and the catchy infomercials. I used to be an insomniac (thank God for curing

me from that), but I would stay up all night

watching infomercials and some Barbie

looking woman would prance on TV and

talk about how in 6 short weeks I could

look like them. If I did what they did. And

for the super low price of $199 or six

instalments of $19.99.

But if I acted right down it would only be 5

instalments. Why not? What did I have to

lose, and they would express ship it to

me. So, I would wait with baited breath for

the mail to come so I could start the road

to skinny! The VHS tape would come and

I would be so excited and start to watch

the tape and a week later back to

business as usual. So, that gimmick didn't

get me skinny, but they would get my

money, so I would move onto the next

thing. And convince myself I was fine.

Name a gym in the northwest Baltimore

Region and I have probably joined it. I

realized I enjoyed group fitness way

better than working out to a tape. It was

the accountability. I needed someone

anticipating my arrival to their class. My

friends in the class would be cheering me

on as I did a move whether it was right

or wrong. I went to gyms off and on for years, but I never reached the desired weight loss that I wanted, and I was always curious as to why. I talked to my co-workers and they would say weight loss was 80% of what you eat and 20% of working out.

Ok so we created these food tracking manuals to record what we ate. But that lasted a hot minute and eating healthy ceased.

So, a friend told me about a weight loss doctor in Essex, MD about how she lost 25 pounds in 3 months. What! Where! Sign

me up! The next week I had an

appointment and the nurse practitioner

was prescribing me phentermine and

another drug neither of which weren't

covered by my insurance but baby when I

tell you I was tight and right! I slimmed

down quickly and in 2007 I was a size 10!

Eureka, I caught the skinny! I loved how my

clothes fit and how I looked. But I didn't like

the dry mouth, dizziness, constipation and the

myriad of other side effects from the drugs I

was ingesting. After hearing about the

baseball player's death caused by

phentermine and finding a lump in my

breast, I stopped taking the pills and the weight came back with a vengeance. I weighed more than I did when I started, I lost the skinny! So, I decided to join yet another gym in 2010 because I wanted my size 10 back but when I didn't see my desired results. I went back to that weight loss clinic and double down on the pills. I knew it was going to work this time because as opposed to just stopping the pills suddenly, I was going to slowly wean myself off the pills and the nurse helped me will an exit strategy. From January to May, I was on the pills and got down to 160 pounds, size 8. You couldn't tell me **ish!** I was the sandwich, chips, pickle, tea and the tray! I was everything because I had reached my definition of skinny. My BMI even told me I was IT! So, once I reached my target weight, I started to reduce my intake of the drugs and proud to grab a size 8 off the racks and size medium shirt. I even had a pair of jeans that was a size 28 waist. Yes, you read that correctly 28-inch waist. I loved it and all the while I was eating what I wanted. I believed it was healthy... maybe some fried chicken here and there and a cheesesteak every now and again.

I ate salads regularly. But when I stopped

the drugs, what happened? You guessed

it. The weight came back, the type of

drugs I was taking I knew they weren't

healthy, but it didn't matter because I was

chasing the skinny! So, from there I

worked out with guys who claimed they

were Personal Trainers. Their

methodology did not help to get to my

achieve goal. I even tried pills certified

by a famous doctor with their own TV

show. But they were nasty, and I didn't

see results fast enough. When a new fad

diet came out, the Skinny Tea, I was on it.

The tea was deplorable and had me in

the bathroom at all ungodly hours. I would

lose a few pounds, but nothing

sustainable over any course of time. After

the tea, I tried to wrap my skinny away. I

was wrapped and trapped and my

friends were having a wrap parties to

instantly lose inches of my waist. Another

fad with no longevity. Money wasted in

all these different scams but I was farther

than ever from my goal.

In 2016, two of my close friends and I

decided this would be the year we were

getting skinny, so we enrolled into a

fitness program that we committed to

working out 2-3 times a week. We

coordinated schedules and became

accountability partners to each other. We

had monthly weigh ins and my weight

was increasing going up. I couldn't

understand it. I was working out, getting

stronger why was the skinny escaping

me. It wasn't until 2017 that I figured out

the secret to my weight loss...

"Mistakes are the portals of
discovery."

-James Joyce

Chapter 2

Eureka!

March 2017, I went to a high school basketball tournament with a couple of family members and ran into a photographer I knew from other events. He asked if he could take a picture of this dynamic trio and we quickly obliged. He sent us the photo and while it was a beautiful picture of the 3 of us. I looked at myself and couldn't believe how big I had become. I knew I struggled to pull on my size 14 jeans and was wearing XL tops, but it hadn't dawned on me I was the size I was. I

knew I had gained a few extra pounds,

but hadn't everyone? I thought it was the

natural progression of life to pack on a few.

But, staring at that picture was the harsh

reality that my weight was out of control and I

had to do something about it. Friends and

family would say things like "Since you're

tall, the weight isn't really noticeable, or it

didn't matter because I was well

proportioned. As it turns out, it did matter to

me and when I finally faced myself, I knew I

had to change.

Like Michael Jackson sang "I'm starting with

the man in the mirror I'm asking myself to

change his ways. No message could have been any clearer if you want to make the world a better place has to look at yourself and make a change." It was at this point my mindset shifted. I wanted to change for myself, and I wanted to document that change so, I could assist others with their transformations.

Women today are not loving their best lives due to issues with their weight and have things holding them back and it's because of their weight… I went back to the gym, but from previous experience I knew the gym alone wasn't going to get me to skinny.

My job had a wellness fair to highlight the

health benefits they had to offer. I went

through the basics, getting my blood drawn

and blood pressure checked, and then my

attention was drawn to the Wellness

Company. I was instantly curious. What is

that? that caught my eye! If you were over 31

BMI which is considered obese you qualified

for the program. I wasn't exactly sure where I

was on the scale but confident it was high

based on that infamous impromptu family

photo. Upon leaving the wellness fair, I went

home, did my research, and found the

program to be reputable and effective. It was

covered by my insurance so there was no out

of pocket cash Great! What did I have to lose

expect the weight? I had seemingly tried

every diet fad and scam out there, with no

lasting results, so why not give this new

program a shot?

It wasn't until April 2017, after what felt like

a lifetime of chasing the skinny, did I discover

the secret. There is no magic pill or formula to

weight loss, there is a mindset shift that has

to occur. I wanted to lose weight but my

approach about it had been all wrong. I would

work out until the cows came home but did

not see significant difference... heck, any

difference... in my waistline. I had to have the

winning combo of eating right, working out

and consistency in order to achieve the desired results. My view of weight loss was distorted as a result of my previous experiences. I thought if I drank this tea for six weeks I would be skinny, or if I wrapped my stomach the fat would magically melt away. It wasn't until I grasped the concept hard work and consistency that I begin to change. I am an adjunct faculty member, so I have taught students about reaching goals. I have set and achieved personal/professional goals in my life. I always had a desire to lose weight but never put a plan into action which included setting goals to achieve it. In April, I enrolled in a weight loss program, this is a 2-

year program for people with a

BMI of 30 or higher. At this time, I was the

largest I have even been at 240lbs. This

comprehensive weight loss program that

tracks eating habits, establishes an exercise

regimen, and focuses on a weekly lesson.

It started with an introductory call from a

health coach. We discussed the program in

depth and what goals I wanted to accomplish.

Never had I mapped out a specific plan to lose

weight. As the weeks went on, we discussed

my food options, exercise weekly, exercise

goals were set, and I would accomplish them.

The food tracking was the area I struggled.

My mindset had to shift. I had to go from the

thought weight loss was going to happen to

to actively engaging in this weight loss

process. If you think it, you can achieve it. I

had to not only believe I was going to lose the

weight but actively lose it by making better

food choices and working out consistently.

I had my first appointment with Health Coach

the first of April. She explained the program

to me and how it

tracked my eating habits and work outs. Once

a week, I would need to weigh myself and

read the learning focus. I learned how to reach

the skinny while having these weekly

conversations with her for the first twelve weeks. I would go on to consistently stick with the program for 2 years. End result: Become a member of a National Weight Loss Registry for those who had lost weight and continued to keep it off for two years. I have been able to be consistent in several areas of my life, but weight loss was not one. One of my strengthens has always been my ability to get assistance when I need it, without allowing fear to get in my way. While utilizing the resources provided by the Health Coach, I was able to witness the transformation in a way that I had never been exposed to before. One thing the coach would constantly emphasize was the importance of my role in all of this. While I had amazing support, it was I who was making the changes and the coach helped me to be proud of that. I had unlocked the mystery.

"Once your mindset changes,
everything on the outside will
change along with it."
-Steve Maraboli

Chapter 3
Mindset Shift

To begin my transformation and reach my goals it all started with my mind. My mind had to envision my goal and lead me to make the change when I lost the weight. Previously, I had wrong intentions. I wanted to lose the weight to fit in this outfit or impress this guy, but never to be healthy. I wanted to fit the image society said I should be. I wanted to compete with supermodels and movie stars. Society does a great job of making girls/women feel they aren't enough and they need to fit into this mold of what a woman should look like. That is why girls are left with low self-esteem and never feeling they are enough but that is another book. Back to me, so within the first couple of weeks I quickly realized my mindset would guide me to my transformation goals. I have accomplished major milestones in my life before and the way I did it was by first envisioning the desired outcome. Graduating summa Cum Laude from A&T and a 3.8 with my master's degree I always remembered my why. When I was pressed against a wall with a deadline or procrastinated until the last minute to get an assignment done I remembered my why and that made me dig a little bit deeper to get it done. So, if I accomplished these majors' feats with remembering my why, couldn't I transfer these skills to the Skinny? Of course, I had to change how I viewed weight loss understand my weight and propel myself to reaching it. Everything starts in your mind; a thought turns into an action. There are so many clichés surrounding it, believe and you can conceive it. There are so many, and they are true. I had to prepare my mind to be a better me. I had to be able to transform my mindset regarding weight loss. I was trying to capture the skinny but not transform my mind that's why I could never sustain the weight lost. My mind had to change who I was and what I was doing. When people would bring up the weight lost and ask if I was on a diet I would quickly correct them and say I'm transforming my lifestyle. A diet is a temporary fix to a permanent problem, like putting a Band-Aid on a gaping hole. Women will diet to fit in a dress or for an upcoming photo shoot. I would lose weight to capture the skinny. That is something that isn't attainable because what is skinny is different to different people an image a concept that is never really achieved. Some people feel skinny is a size 4 to 10 so essentially, I was chasing something that could never be mine. That's why I had to shift my mindset. I was trying to have a healthy lifestyle once I understood that concept and set in my mind the pounds came off. Wouldn't the world be a better place if all you had to do was change your mind and the weight melts off. Of course, then we would all be at our weight goals. The mindset shift was accompanied with changing my eating habits, ramping up my exercise regimen and the dreaded C

word...Consistency!

"You are what you eat, so don't be Fast, Cheap, Easy or Fake"

-Unknown

Chapter 4
Eating Right

The journey of 1,000 miles begins with one step. Signing up for a health coach was that first step for me! One component of the program was tracking what I ate. My daily caloric intake for my BMI, is 1,500 calories or less. Never had I been a calorie counter, but I always thought I ate relatively healthy. I had a salad occasionally. I would get a flour tortilla

wrap and thought that was good for me.
For the past 20 years on and off I was
chasing the skinny and trying to get to a
certain size and thought if I ate well and
worked out I would achieve that goal. That
so wasn't the case! I heard people would
say weight lost was 80/20. 80% what you
ate and 20% of what you did (exercise).
Well I thought I was doing that, but the
weight was not coming off. When I was in
hot pursuit of the skinny, the supplement
along with exercise made the scale move.
Several years passed before I realized that
what I was eating was making all the
difference. When I started to track what I

ate, I came very quickly to the realization that I ate horribly! One evening I ate four slices of pizza, which by themselves took me over my allotted calories, not to mention the breakfast and lunch I had consumed earlier that day. I thought salad was healthy but the way I fixed them they would total 1,000 calories 2/3 of my expected daily intake. Even an after-work trip to happy hour resulted in excess calorie consumption. Anyone that knows me knows I'm a candy addict. My favorite holidays were November 1, December 26 and February 15 because they were the days after the major holidays and candy was 50% off. I would rather snack on candy than eat real food any day. If it was a new candy on the market I was the unofficial taste tester trying it out and giving my friends, my unsolicited opinion.

A turning point for me was when I decided to participate in a friend's " No Sweets" challenge. For the entire month of April, I made the commitment to give up cakes, candy, cookies, and pies. Day 1 was smoother than expected and I kept focusing on what I wanted. In order to achieve something different, I had to be willing to change my plan of action. By Day 5, I was experiencing real and severe withdrawals that clearly showed me just how intense my addiction to sweets really was. It was time to cut ties with this toxic relationship. I reflected on my goals to regain the strength to forge ahead. To satisfy the craving for sugar, I would eat more fruits and vegetables. Within the first two weeks, I was amazed to see and feel results. I was much more energized and even started attending a 6am yoga class. I **started to eat more fruit and vegetables and less sweets,** Also, the removal of sweets caused a reduction in my calorie intake and resulted in noticeable weight loss. Once I maintained control of my calorie consumption and increased my physical activity, the pounds seemed to fall off. I was feeling great and it was important to me to continue to progress. In May, I made the decision to also cut out bread, pasta, rice, and potatoes. Being a bread lover, this would also be a huge challenge, but I was so determined that I was willing to endure the hard parts. Even when dining at my favorite restaurants, I would simply turn down any offers of specialty rolls while my friends indulged and I would sip my water. Temptation is something serious and I made the choice to remain steadfast in my quest to catch the skinny.

By trade I'm an event planner, so I knew the best way to reach my goals was to plan, and that's when I started to meal prep, I would go to the store on Sunday and purchase what I would eat for the week. Do you know there are so many benefits with meal prepping? It saves money, first of all. Buying in bulk, rather than eating out every day or purchasing individual meals, was a smart choice for me. Those dollars here and there had been adding up! It saves money. You don't have to think about what you will eat. I would make bad food choices by going too fast food restaurants and picking up food because I was hungry, with meal prep I didn't have to worry because I knew exactly what I was going to eat. I would plan down to the snacks what I was going to eat I didn't want to leave my food option to questions. I would prep 2-3 options for breakfast. 2-3 different sandwiches for lunch, 2-3 vegetables/fruit options, 2-3 meats, 2 starches for dinner.

A typical day might consist of the following:

Breakfast: Boiled egg, ½ grapefruit, 2 sausage links

Snack: Green apple and 2 tablespoons of peanut butter

Lunch: Chicken Southwest salad

Snack: Celery and Cucumbers

Dinner: 4 oz Chicken Breast, Small Baked Potato, Steamed Broccoli and Carrots

With meal prep I was dropping the weight consistently, and still eating the foods I loved.

Another drastic change to my nutrition regimen involved beverages. I went from drinking soda, juice, tea, and alcohol, to

ONLY consuming water. Like many people, I

never once realized just how many calories

beverages accounted for. I was living under

the common misconception that the 1,500

calories a day diet was strictly about food and

had little or nothing to do with drinks. For

example, if you have an orange juice for

breakfast that's 250 calories, sweet tea for

lunch is another 280 calories, and a 16 oz

soda for dinner is responsible for an

additional 150 calories. That's a whopping

680 calories, leaving you only 820 calories to consume for food. Don't get me started on alcohol. I used to be a social drinker. I'd have a cocktail or two at happy hour, or at a friend's house. I loved a wine fest! I would leave with bottles to enjoy. A five-ounce serving of white wine (my fav) is 120 calories and I don't know about you, but I could throw back several glasses of wine. Giving up drinks and alcohol was a huge step for me, but I knew if I wanted to reach my goal, it had to be done. For those who are already shaking

their heads, not able to imagine giving up that

oh-so-necessary wine, let me introduce you to

an awesome word: Moderation. If you know

you are going to a happy hour, perhaps cut out

your afternoon snack and enjoy ONE glass of

wine. While out with your friends, consider

ordering water for you to also enjoy once you

have finished that delicious glass of wine.

Most bars have fancy waters you can

purchase if you still want to look trendy. Like

me, you will quickly learn that water is filling

and results in a decrease in your food

consumption. By drinking 20 oz of water at

every meal, I was able to maintain my target

intake every day. Only drinking water, the

pounds started to leave my body and my waist

started to shrink.

"Good things come to those who sweat."

-Unknown

Chapter 5

Work, Work, Work

I love to dance! When I went to the club, I was often the first person on the floor and the last to leave. I would come alive on the dance floor; the music would speak to my soul and that's where I wanted to stay. As a child, I participated in ballet, modern dance and cheerleading, I was always jumping around so my mom put that rambunctious energy into constructive activity. As life went on, I held onto the passion for dance; however, I lacked the energy to participate in it on a regular basis.

In my pursuit for the skinny I would buy exercise DVDs from those persuasive infomercials to work out at home. (VHS tapes but I'm dating myself.) I would start with all the vigorous energy and dance to the beat but would never sustain it for a long period of time. I even joined several gyms and would take group classes. There, I learned the accountability that came from group exercise. My work out buddies would look for me, the instructors knew my name and would question when I was missing. I loved it, but unless I was taking the supplement would not see the scale move. It was so frustrating and eventually I stopped going. I felt like a hamster in a wheel, running but not getting anywhere.

The milestone year of turning 40 I was tired of being tired. I had grown weary of feeling like I did not have enough energy to do anything. I would go to work, go home, sleep occasionally go out, but felt like I was tired all the time. I talked to a few friends and we all enrolled in a fitness program. I knew instantly that this time I would go to the distance. The program had clear expectations. I was to work out 2 - 3 times a week and be open to advisement from a fitness coach in regard to which classes I needed to take. I had a busy schedule with working multiple jobs so only certain classes would fit into my schedule. I knew from previous experience with group fitness classes that I would attend as long as I was having a good time. My coach recommended a class called MixxedFit®. I had never heard of it, and she explained it was a people inspired fitness program that is a mix of explosive dancing and boot camp toning. The first time I took the class it was an instant love affair. We danced to songs on the radio and I could not get enough of the classes. I took every class I could! There was a feeling that came over me when the beat dropped, and it held onto me the entire class. The fitness studio owner pointed out how good I was and thought I should consider becoming an instructor.

Although I was passionate about dancing and music, I hadn't once considered being a fitness instructor. But, she believed in me and encouraged me to believe in myself, so I took her suggestion and ran with it. I trained for the next few months preparing for the workshop.

MixxedFit® choreography is a combination of easy repetitive moves to songs heard on the radio so the participants can focus on maximizing their workouts effectively and not focus on complicated choreography. The training was 8 hours with an audition at the conclusion to determine who became instructors. The MixxedFit® community was so supportive. Once the other instructors found out my intentions, they worked with me to ensure I became an instructor. They let me lead songs in their classes and even stayed after class to help me. They were really rooting for me to succeed. The life changing day consisted of an 8-hour gruelling process, something I was not used to at this level. But 80% of success is showing up, so I was there and determined to become an instructor. At the end of the day I was victorious and now a Licensed MixxedFit® Instructor. At the age of 40 I was "over the moon' proud of myself and learned it is never too late to accomplish my dreams. I believed therefore, I achieved.

By no means am I advising you to become an instructor to get in shape. I'm relaying the path I took. What I would advise is figure out what works best for you. If you like to ride a bicycle than do that as your form of exercise. If you are an early bird and your gym offers morning classes, attend the 6am boot camp. Order that DVD reduced 50% from that late-night infomercial and work out regularly to it. I knew group exercise was fun for me since I'm a social person who also needs accountability factor. MixxedFit® was the right "fit" for me but I didn't limit myself to that format. I loved the serenity yoga offered, it was my one-hour oasis. I was able to relax, deep breath and stretch my muscles. My gym only offered it 6am and I'm far from a morning person but the energy boost I had acquired since breaking up with sweets made it easier to participate in those classes.

Gyms offer a wide variety of group fitness classes, equipment, and 1:1 personal trainer. First, figure out what works for you, then do it consistently.

"Consistency isn't rocket
science, it's commitment."
-Mattieologie

Chapter 6

Is that a 4-letter word?

Consistency is often the equivalent of the

nastiest of the four-letter words! It's great to

eat one clean meal or have one killer workout

but the only way to lose the weight is to do

those things over a sustained amount of time.

Many times, people know exactly what to do

to achieve their goal. If I want to buy a new

car, I need to have a decent credit score and

save or have money for a down payment. If I

want a better job, I have to apply, and

possibly obtain additional skills, which may require me to go back to school. When developing a title for this book I was going to title it The Secret of my Weight Loss but the reality is there is no secret! To achieve weight loss, you have to make better food choices, work out and maintain consistency. So why don't people do it when they know exactly what has to be done? For most of us, everything depends on when and if they have that aha! or rock bottom moment. My aha! was when I realized I was a human yo-yo with my weight. My rock bottom was when I has exceeded my "scary" weight by 40 pounds. I was ready to set new goals and create new habits. When I didn't feel like

going to the gym, I would remind myself of

the goals I had set, I would look at that picture

from March 2017 because I knew I never

wanted to be that woman again. It takes 30

days to form a habit… 30 days. Constantly, I

denied myself what I loved in search for a

better future. Do I eat candy now? Yeah,

occasionally but nowhere near how I used to.

I don't go candy shopping the day after

holidays to rack up on candy. I learned how to

eat it in moderation and that aligns with my

new goals. Every once in a while, I may have

a slice of pizza… but not four! I might skip a

workout for a day…but not a week. I traded

my old lifestyle for a healthier one, complete

with clean eating and a regimen of physical

activities… all catered to meet my needs.

What will be your constant? Only you can

answer that for yourself. Do you go to work

multiple days a week? If so, what's your

motivation since you haven't been doing that

consistently over a long period of time? You

have to apply those same principles to

develop consistency for your new lifestyle. I

struggled with consistency for years. Not just

in weight loss, but life in general I would start

a project and not finish. I would begin a task,

only to abandon it for another item on my

agenda. People in my life would point it out

and I would brush it off and never

acknowledge my flaw. As I approached this

journey I had to fully acknowledge who I

was, where I wanted to go and maintain the

belief I was going to get there. What was I

going to do to make things different this time?

I had to make this journey fit me and not fit

the journey. I had to discover food I like and

would be able to sustain me for a long period

of time. Try different fruits and vegetables.

Eat veggie noodles instead of linguini.

Experiment with different recipes. The

internet is filled with healthy food options.

Just a little research and motivation is all it

takes. Eating what I like has afforded me the

opportunity to continue on my healthy

journey. Figure out what exercise format

works for you and you will be able to stay

constant.

Consistency is the key for any sustainable

change in your life.

"You are allowed to be a
masterpiece and work in progress
simultaneously."
-Unknown

Chapter 7

End of the Road not really but end of this book

At the beginning of my fitness journey, I was Chasing the Skinny... running after something that never truly existed. It was Society's construct of an image that was unattainable.

In the end, I did find a healthy version of myself. I learned to love myself for exactly who I was. It was all about self-evaluation, reflection and making changes for myself and

nobody else. I discovered I could continue to

eat what I wanted and become the size I

wanted to be. Fad diets are just that. A fad,

passing trend and have temporary results. I

discovered the vital combination of eating

healthy and exercise over a long period

of time as a healthy means to lose weight and

maintain a healthier lifestyle. If you have been

sedentary in your lifestyle, don't attempt to

exercise 5 days a week. Start with 1-2 days

for twenty minutes. Group classes are great

but listen to your body and if you are getting

overheated, slow down. There is no shame in

being unable to finish a class, you'll get there.

Move at your own pace to avoid being

overwhelmed and running the risk of quitting.

Remember, you are not in competition with

anyone else because they aren't running your

race.

Building your body's exercise tolerance could

and should take some time. Before you know

it you will increase the number of days you

are working out. The plan only works if you

work it.

Hope this book has given YOU the insight

and strength YOU need to inspire the change

YOU seek.

Thank you allowing me to my journey! I

wish you success and positive vibes as you

embark on yours!

If you can't get enough of *Chasing the Skinny*, please check out my website: **www.chasingtheskinny.com** where you will find Chasing the Skinny merchandise and Chasing the Skinny Meal Prep programs. Start your weight loss journey utilizing my services to ensure you reach your goals.